50 Fat Busting Juicing Recipes

Great Weight Loss and Detox Recipes

By: Amy Zulpa

TABLE OF CONTENTS

Publishers Notes 3

Dedication 4

Chapter 1- What Is Juicing and What Are the Advantages? 5

Chapter 2- Is Juicing for Everyone? 10

Chapter 3- 10 Fat Busting Fruit Juice Recipes 14

Chapter 4- 10 Fat Busting Green Juice Recipes 22

Chapter 5- 10 Fat Busting Smoothie Recipes 29

Chapter 6- 10 Fat Busting Fruit & Juice Recipes 36

Chapter 7- 10 Fat Busting Detox Juice Recipes 45

About the Author 53

Publishers Notes

Disclaimer

This publication is intended to provide helpful and informative material. It is not intended to diagnose, treat, cure, or prevent any health problem or condition, nor is intended to replace the advice of a physician. No action should be taken solely on the contents of this book. Always consult your physician or qualified health-care professional on any matters regarding your health and before adopting any suggestions in this book or drawing inferences from it.

The author and publisher specifically disclaim all responsibility for any liability, loss or risk, personal or otherwise, which is incurred as a consequence, directly or indirectly, from the use or application of any contents of this book.

Any and all product names referenced within this book are the trademarks of their respective owners. None of these owners have sponsored, authorized, endorsed, or approved this book.

Always read all information provided by the manufacturers' product labels before using their products. The author and publisher are not responsible for claims made by manufacturers.

© 2014

Manufactured in the United States of America

DEDICATION

This book is dedicated to all those people who seek health and wellness. The journey can be difficult but it does pay off in the long run.

Chapter 1 - What Is Juicing and What Are the Advantages?

Juicing is the newest craze in dieting. Just like Atkins, Paleo, and South Beach diets in the past, juicing has become the latest popular diet, even with celebrities. Juicing is used to lose weight and cleanse the body of toxins while avoiding solid foods for a period of time which is usually a few days to several weeks. The juice is derived from whole fruits and vegetables which are then blended to reduce the ingredients into a liquid juice.

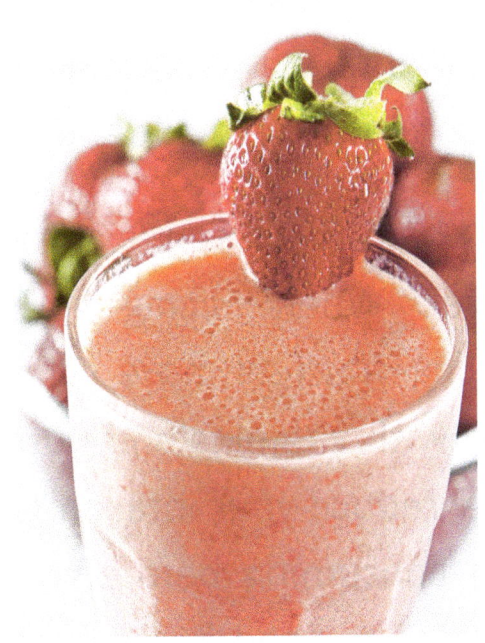

A typical juice is made mostly from greens with other fruits and veggies added. It can consist of a blend of kale, broccoli, green apples, collard greens, spinach, or coconut water. The juice used for juicing is specially made, not usually bought in a supermarket. Most juices in the supermarket contain lots of added sugars, and they do not provide the same benefit as having freshly juiced whole fruits and veggies.

Not only is juicing beneficial for those who want to lose weight but it can also provide much needed vitamins and nutrients to your diet that may have been lacking. It can also help eliminate the consumption of processed foods and sugars, can act as a healthy meal replacement, is healthier for you than store bought juices, is easier to absorb nutrients from than solid foods, and it can also give your digestive system a little rest. The benefits to juicing, outside of the increase of nutrients and decrease in toxins are that it will help your body have a regulated colon, increase your energy and stamina, regulate your sleep patterns for the better, increase your mental clarity, and leave you with a glowing complexion in addition to healthy nails and hair.

Juicing is designed to help you lose weight and eliminate certain foods from your diet. When juicing your appetite becomes reduced just by making you feel more satisfied since your food intake is now packed with vitamins and nutrients. Just by juicing you will automatically reduce your intake of damaging foods that you may have been consuming before. Many people have an intolerance or sensitivity to food items such as dairy, toxic fats, gluten, wheat, processed sugar, and other additives. Since juicing is the product of raw fruits and vegetables, all the harmful additives are gone from your diet. Not only will this make you feel physically better but it can help identify which foods your body is intolerant to by reintroducing them slowly after your cleanse is complete.

The juice is loaded with things that are good for your body- such as vitamins, minerals, anti-inflammatory components, and antioxidants. These nutrients you are flooding your body with can help protect you against cardiovascular disease, cancer, and rheumatoid arthritis. Juicing also provides a way to get the daily recommended amounts of fruits and vegetables, especially if you are not a fan of certain whole fruits and veggies. By juicing the fruits and veggies instead of cooking you are still receiving the nutrients that you would in the raw, whole food which would otherwise be destroyed if cooked. These nutrients in the raw fruits and veggies help your body digest easier and provide anti-inflammatory enzymes.

Juicing works to detox your body by allowing some of your major digestive organs- your stomach, intestines, and liver, to rest for the period you are consuming the nutrient packed juice. It can take your body up to 18 hours to digest and remove just one meal which can require your digestive system to work non-stop sometimes, depending on your food intake. Juice requires less stomach acid to digest which can reduce the need for acid reducing medications. Foods that are heavy in refined carbs, saturated fats, and additives are harsh on your intestines and can cause stress on them which will impair certain functions.

These foods upset the delicate balance in your intestines and can even cause breaks in your intestinal linings or barriers. Digesting the juice requires less energy on your intestines, giving them a much needed break and time to rest and repair. Juicing requires less stress and consumes less energy when being digested by the intestines. The liver is the organ that handles detoxification in the body. When food is absorbed into the intestines it then moves into the liver to detoxify and entering the rest of your body. Many processed foods contain so many toxins that the liver is overworked. Juicing will give your liver a chance to take a break and become less overwhelmed.

Health benefits aside, juicing can just make you feel better overall. Juicing will improve your energy supply without the need for caffeine or stimulants. Chronic physical issues such as headaches, bloating, excess gas, rashes, and congestion should being to clear when flooding your body with vitamins and nutrients during juicing. Many people consume liquids outside of water like sodas, coffee, tea, or alcohol. Juicing will rehydrate your body and speed up the process of eliminating toxins. A mentioned beforehand, the influx of nutrients, vitamins will also add a sheen to your hair and nails, while reducing any redness to the skin. Juicing with raw fruits and veggies can leave you feeling more refreshed and energized than any caffeine drink could leave you feeling!

The benefits of juicing are many, which is no wonder why it is the latest craze in dieting! Just by purchasing your own juicer and a variety of whole, raw fruits and vegetables you can begin juicing as well. Juicing will leave you seeing and feeling results such as weight loss, improved energy, stamina, and mental clarity, and leave you feeling radiant and rejuvenated!

CHAPTER 2- IS JUICING FOR EVERYONE?

If you have heard a lot of your friends and family talk about juicing, you might find yourself wondering if that is something you should be looking into. However, you might have stopped yourself from looking too much into it because you are afraid that it will take a lot of work or cost a lot of money. This is hardly the case and once you learn what it is all about, you will be very interested in making sure that you are giving juicing a try.

The Health Benefits

As mentioned in chapter one, the main reason people will start juicing is that they get a lot of health benefits from it. You know what you are putting in the juicer. You also know that you are not adding any additives or preservatives that store bought juices contain. This means that you are creating the best juice for you and your family. The juice that you will make will be packed full of vitamins and minerals. It will also be extremely fresh, which is the best way to drink your juice if you want to make sure that you are getting the most out of it.

When you start juicing on a regular basis, you will find that you will start to feel better overall. You will sleep better and your skin will begin to look and feel better. Many people have reported that after juicing for just a short time that they find themselves with a lot of energy that they have needed for so long. This makes working out and tending to the everyday chores around the house or yard a lot easier to deal with.

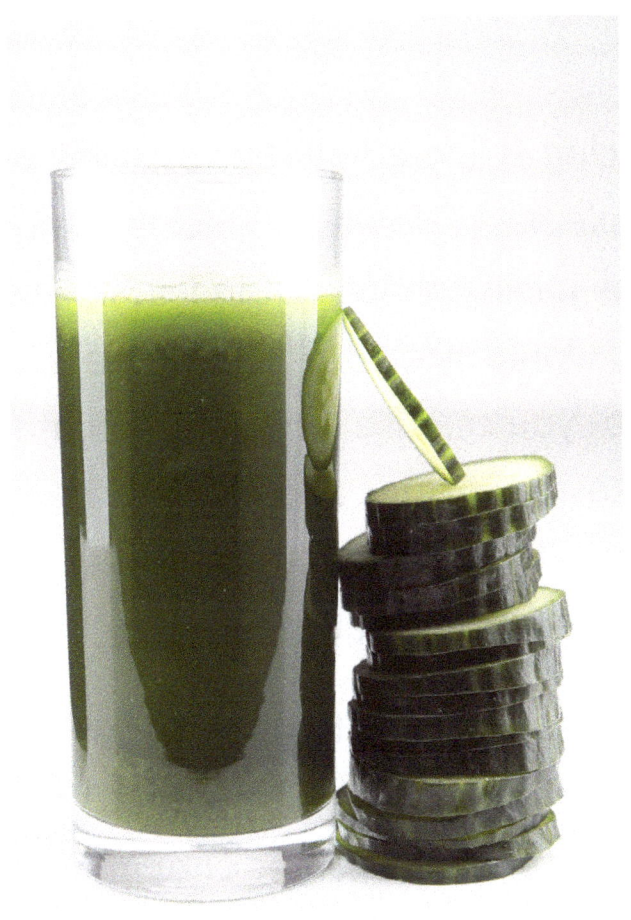

Do You Have To Buy An Expensive Machine?

If you are worried that you are going to have to purchase a super expensive juicer in order to make this work, worry no more. Sure, there are some very high-tech juicers out there that can cost hundreds of dollars, but you really do not have to pay that much. You can easily find a relatively inexpensive juicer for around forty dollars at many local department stores. You should also have no trouble find a few great options for juicers online. Just make sure that you are doing your best to purchase a juicer that comes with a good warranty. This way, no matter how much you are spending, your investment in the juicer is well protected.

How Hard Is It?

Thinking that juicing is incredibly hard is one of the things that hold a lot of people back. However, juicing really is not that hard. All you need is a juicing machine and a selection of fruits and veggies that you would like to use. There are a wide variety of recipes online that you can use or you can create your own. Many people will take tested recipes and make it their own by adding a little something to it. Others will simply use whatever leftover fruit they have in their refrigerator and juice that.

Simply plug in your juicer and then cut up the pieces of fruit or veggies you want to use and start putting it through the juicer. It may take a couple of minutes to get enough juice for a glass, but you will be thrilled with the effort when you taste how incredible your juice is. A good tip to remember is that you will want to clean your juicer immediately in order to prevent bits and pieces of dried food from clogging up the machine – making it almost impossible to clean.

How Much Does It Really Cost?

The amount you will spend on juicing will have a lot to do with how you approach it. Some people go to the store to purchase food specifically for the juicer. Others will buy from local farm stands or even grow their own in order to save money. Then you have the people that do not juice regularly, and simply make use of whatever they have in the house when they are ready to do a little juicing. How often you juice, how many people you are juicing for, and what types of fruits and veggies you will use will determine the actual cost of the juicing.

Some people find that they are able to save a lot of money while others find they spend more in comparison to what they could have purchased from the store. However, the health benefits and the exceptional taste certainly make the entire cost and process of juicing well worth it. Whether you are juicing regularly for a special diet or simply doing it when the urge strikes you, this is something that you will want to give a try.

Give It a Try

Exploring all of the different juicing recipes that you can find will be a lot of fun for the entire family. Many people find that they even have a blast creating their own juicing recipe from scratch. Will this be something that you end up wanting to do on a regular basis? Maybe or maybe not. Juicing everyday may not be for everyone, but it is almost impossible to find anyone that has said that they do not enjoy the occasional fresh made juice. Simply give it a try for yourself. Don't give up if your first recipe does not pan out the way you wanted for it to. Keep trying a few different options while you discover what works best for your budget and taste buds.

CHAPTER 3- 10 FAT BUSTING FRUIT JUICE RECIPES

Juicing has become exceptionally popular with those that are looking to lose weight. Many fruits and vegetables contain minerals that aid in burning fat. Juicing is undoubtedly the way to go considering that cooking foods destroy some of their micronutrients. Processed foods usually lack some of their micronutrients also. In order to get the maximum nutrition value from your fruits and vegetables, juicing is the best option as well as buying only organic products when able. Juicing also helps you get your daily recommended servings of fruits and vegetables in your diet easily. These juices are not only effective in burning fat but are tasty! Far more than one aspect of juicing greatly contributes to your weight loss success. Making your own juices is most certainly something worth trying; but how do you make them? No worries, we've got you covered. We've gathered up 10 delicious fat busting fruit juice recipes to help get you started.

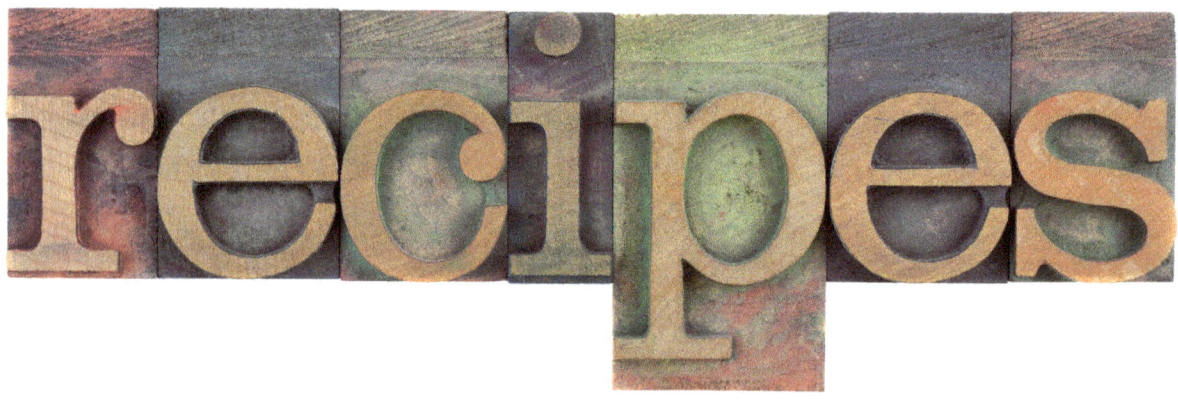

Papaya Passion

This tropical flavored juice is loaded with vitamin C, which plays a big role in weight loss. Papayas also contain papain, an enzyme that helps with digestion and contributes to the breaking down of proteins.

Ingredients

1 medium papaya
1 red Apple
5 pitted dates

Directions

Remove stem from apple and papaya if applicable. Place all three ingredients in a blender

Blend well and serve fresh

Strawberry Delight

This juice will help give you an energy boost. Strawberries are great for breaking down carbohydrates. Dates are beneficial because of their natural fibers that keep you feeling full. They are also a good source of protein, various minerals and numerous vitamins, including vitamin C. Dates contain natural sugars that make them great energy boosters.

Ingredients

5-8 strawberries
1-2 bananas
9-10 pitted dates

Directions

Peel bananas. Remove the tops of the strawberries

Place all three ingredients in a blender. Blend well and serve fresh

A Taste of Heaven

This refreshing juice provides you with many health benefits to help burn fat. The fruits in this juice each provide you with their own benefits regarding vitamins and minerals. Dulse is scientifically proven to be an antioxidant. Dulse is also very rich in protein, iodine and potassium.

Ingredients

5-6 blueberries
4 strawberries
2 apples
3-4 pitted dates
Pinch of dulse powder

Directions

Remove stems from the apples. Place all ingredients in a blender.

Blend well and serve fresh.

Watermelon Juice

This delicious juice is perfect for burning fat. Watermelon contains arginine. Arginine is an amino acid that both prevents the storing of fat and burns it.

Ingredients

½ of a seedless watermelon
½ cup of coconut water
1 lime
Pinch of cayenne pepper

Directions

Peel and chop up watermelon into chunks. Place the seedless watermelon, coconut water and cayenne pepper in a blender.

Cut the lime in half. Squeeze the juice from one half of the lime into the blender.

Blend well and serve fresh

Slim Me Juice

This juice is excellent for weight loss. This juice boosts metabolism and increases stamina during exercise.

Ingredients

1 apple
4-5 raspberries

1 kiwi

1 banana

4 almonds

Directions

Remove stem from apple. Peel banana. Place all ingredients in a blender

Blend and serve fresh

Tropical Green Tea Power

This juice is great for energy and is protein-rich. Green tea is a powerful antioxidant. Flax seeds contain omega. Bananas and mangos are rich in fiber and vitamins.

Ingredients

½ peeled banana

½ cup mango chunks

1 cup peach juice

1 tbsp. ground flax seeds

1 tbsp. green tea powder

Directions

Place all ingredients in a blender. Blend and serve fresh

Rejuvenating Citrus

This citrus flavored juice is loaded with minerals and vitamins to help you burn fat. The pulp in the orange juice is also loaded with dietary fibers to aid in healthy digestion.

Ingredients

2 apples
5 pineapple slices
8-10 strawberries
½ cup orange juice with pulp

Directions

Place all ingredients in a blender. Blend and serve fresh

Antioxidant Elixir

This juice will keep you feeling full because of its fiber while providing you with a multitude of necessary vitamins and minerals. The Orange juice in this recipe will give you a burst of vitamin c and the green tea has extraordinary antioxidant effects and boosts metabolism.

Ingredients

½ cup orange juice
½ apple
¼ cup pineapple
1 tbsp. green tea powder

Directions

Place all ingredients in a blender. Blend and serve fresh.

Orange Grapefruit Juice

This juice promotes weight loss. Grapefruit is high in fat burning enzymes. Scientific studies have shown many positive connections between drinking grapefruit and weight loss.

Ingredients

3 oranges
1 grapefruit

Directions

Peel the oranges and grapefruit. Place all ingredients in a blender

Blend and serve fresh

Blackberry Grape Goodness

This juice not only helps you burn fat but will also help you to lose water weight by slipping asparagus in the mix. Asparagus is capable of helping you to lose water weight because it is a diuretic. It also has no cholesterol and is low in sodium. Asparagus contains potassium which is widely known for reducing fat. Asparagus is a sugar filler in this recipe and the flavor is overpowered by the blackberries and grapes. Piceatannol, a compound found in grapes and blackberries, helps to stop fat cells from developing and growing.

Amy Zulpa

Ingredients

1 cup blackberries

2 cups red grapes

2 asparagus

Directions

Add all ingredients to a blender

Blend and serve fresh

Chapter 4 - 10 Fat Busting Green Juice Recipes

The advantages of juicing are many, which is no wonder why it has become one of the most popular diets around. Just by purchasing your own juicer and a variety of whole, raw fruits, greens, and vegetables you can be on your way to making your own healthy green, fat busting juices. Consuming green juices will leave you seeing and feeling results such as weight loss, improved energy, stamina, and mental clarity, and leave you feeling healthy and slimmer! You will find below ten recipes to get you started making your own green juices.

Zucchini Power-Up Blast

Ingredients

2 small green zucchinis
½ cup of small green cabbage
2 small green apples
4 green Kale leaves
1 cup of blueberries
1 mango
½ medium cucumber

Directions

Wash all produce. Trim the zucchini ends. Dice the cabbage to fit into the juicer. Quarter apples and discard seeds. Remove any stems from the blueberries. Peel mango and discard seed. Place all produce into your juicer and blend. If you would like to make your green juice a little sweeter, add a 1/3 cup of shredded coconut to the juice. This can be blended with or served over ice if desired. Stir and drink immediately.

Mean Green Machine Juice

Ingredients

1 bunch of Kale
½ bunch of Spinach
2 Celery stalks
2 green apples
1 small bunch of Parsley
2 Carrots

Directions

Wash all produce. Roll kale and spinach into balls to fit into your juicer. Quarter apples and discard seeds. Peel carrots. Place all produce into your juicer and blend. This can be blended with or served over ice if desired. Stir and drink immediately.

Speedy Recovery Juice

Ingredients

4 Kale leaves
½ avocado
1 banana

2 small green apples

2 oranges

½ cup blueberries

Directions

Wash all produce. Roll kale leaves into balls to fit better into the juicer. Halve avocado, remove pit and peel. Peel banana. Quarter apples and discard seeds. Peel oranges and remove all seeds. Remove any stems from the blueberries. Place all produce into your juicer and blend. Add 1/3 cup of shredded coconut for sweetness if desired. This can be blended with or served over ice if desired. Stir and drink immediately.

Afternoon Veggie Delight

Ingredients

2 large broccoli stalks

¼ head of green cabbage

2 celery stalks

¼ head of romaine lettuce

2 green apples

1 orange

2 carrots

Directions

Wash all produce. Chop broccoli, romaine, and cabbage to fit into your juicer. Quarter apples and remove all seeds. Peel orange and carrots. Remove all seeds from the orange. Place all produce into your juicer and blend. This can be blended with or served over ice if desired. Stir and drink immediately.

The Energizer

Ingredients

4 Kale leaves
½ bunch of Spinach
½ bunch of Parsley
2 Celery stalks
⅓ head of Romaine lettuce
2 green apples
1 orange
½ medium cucumber

Directions

Wash all produce. Roll kale and spinach leaves to fit into your juicer. Chop romaine lettuce. Quarter green apples and remove all seeds. Peel orange and remove all seeds. Add all produce into the juicer and blend. This can be blended with or served over ice if desired. Stir and drink immediately.

The Slimmer

Ingredients

½ bunch of Spinach

1 cup of green cabbage
2 celery stalks
½ of a beet
2 green apples
1 cucumber
1 orange

Directions

Wash all produce. Roll spinach leaves to fit into your juicer. Shred cabbage. Quarter green apples and remove all seeds. Peel orange and remove all seeds. Place all ingredients into your juicer and blend. This can be blended with or served over ice if desired. Stir and drink immediately.

The Toxin Blaster

Ingredients

½ bunch of Spinach
4 Kale leaves
3 green apples
1/3 head of Romaine lettuce
2 oranges

Directions

Wash all produce. Roll spinach and kales leaves to fit into your juicer. Quarter green apples and remove all seeds. Chop romaine lettuce. Peel oranges and remove all seeds. Place all produce into your juicer and blend. This can be blended with or served over ice if desired. Stir and drink immediately.

The Morning Power-Up

Ingredients

½ bunch of Spinach
3 Kale leaves
2 green apples
⅓ of a Pineapple
1 orange
½ of a medium cucumber

Directions

Wash all produce. Roll spinach and kale leaves to fit into your juicer. Quarter green apples and remove all seeds. Dice pineapple into small cubes. Peel orange and remove all seeds. Place all produce into your juicer and blend. This can be blended with or served over ice if desired. Stir and drink immediately.

The Green Fruity Punch

Ingredients

2 green apples
3 Kiwi fruits
1/3 of a Pineapple
2 oranges

4 Kale leaves

½ avocado

Directions

Wash all produce. Quarter apples and remove all seeds. Peel kiwis and quarter. Remove skin from the pineapple and cut into chunks. Peel oranges and remove seeds. Roll kale leaves to fit into your juicer. Remove pit and skin from the avocado. Blend all ingredients in your juicer. This can be blended with or served over ice if desired. Stir and drink immediately.

The Hunger Blaster

Ingredients

1 whole Cucumber

2 green apples

3 Celery stalks

2 oranges

½ bunch of Spinach

Directions

Wash all produce. Quarter apples and remove all seeds. Peel oranges and remove all seeds. Roll spinach leaves to fit into your juicer. Blend all produce together in your juicer. This can be blended with or served over ice if desired. Stir and drink immediately.

Chapter 5 - 10 Fat Busting Smoothie Recipes

Keep in mind Smoothies fill up your stomach which keeps you from being hungry for a while.

Oatmeal Fruit Smoothie

Ingredients

½ cup steel-cut oats*
½ cup frozen fruit, such as pineapple or strawberries
½ c. ice cubes
1 packet Stevia**
Ground cinnamon to taste

Directions

Put the oats in the blender and pulse until they reach a powdery consistency. Turn off the blender and add 1 cup water. Incorporate the remaining ingredients into the mix and blend until smooth. Serve

*Steel-cut oats are whole grain groats (the inner portion of the oat kernel) which have been cut into pieces.

**Stevia is a one hundred percent natural sweetener.

Peach and White Bean Smoothie

Ingredients

½ cup unsweetened rice milk

1 cup frozen peaches

¼ cup canned white beans (like cannellini, navy or Great Northern

1/8 teaspoon cinnamon

Pinch of nutmeg

Directions

Pour the rice milk into the blender Add the remaining ingredients and blend until smooth. People who didn't know there were beans in this smoothie couldn't taste them.

Belly Fat Burning Smoothie

Ingredients

½ avocado

¼ cup Greek Yogurt

½ cup of Pomegranate juice

½ tablespoon honey

½ teaspoon vanilla extract

½ cup ice

1 tablespoon Whey Protein*

Directions

Put all ingredients in blender and blend away until your desired smoothness consistency.

*Whey Protein helps build muscle which helps you to burn calories.

Orange and Banana Smoothie (Also a Belly Fat Burning Smoothie)

Ingredients

1 orange
1 banana
1 cup frozen mixed berries
2 Tablespoons Whey Protein
2 Tablespoons Flax Seed
1 cup of ice (optional)

Directions

Put all ingredients in your blender and blend away until you reach your desired consistency of smoothness.

Mixed Berry-Cashew Smoothie

Ingredients

¼ cup raw cashews
½ cup almond milk
1 cup frozen mixed berries

Directions

Grind the raw cashews to a powder in the blender. Add the almond milk, then the berries. Blend until smooth.

Vegan Vanilla Milkshake Smoothie

Ingredients

½ cup soft tofu*
1 cup vanilla soy milkshake
1 frozen banana
½ tablespoon peanut butter

Directions

Mix until smooth.

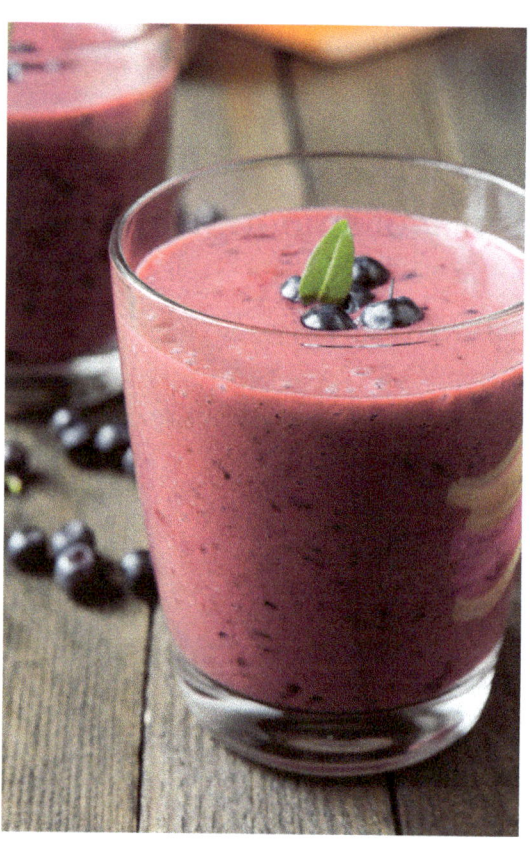

Strawberry and Blueberry Smoothie

Ingredients

1 scoop Whey Protein Strawberry Flavor

40g frozen strawberries

40g frozen blueberries

125g activia vanilla*

200ml water

10g peanut butter

Directions

Blend until smooth and serve.

*Activia vanilla is fat free yogurt.

Mango-Peach Smoothie

Ingredients

2 small champagne mangoes or one large regular mango

1 large peach, pitted

5 ounces fresh baby spinach

4 to 6 ounces of filtered water

Directions

Add all the ingredients to your blender and blend on high for 30 seconds or until creamy.

Green Citrus Smoothie

Ingredients

1 cup spinach

1 orange

1 grapefruit

1 tablespoon honey

3 cups water

Ice

Directions

Blend until consistency is smooth and serve.

Super X Smoothie

Ingredients

1 cup spinach

2 leaves collard greens

1 lime

1-in piece fresh ginger root

½ inch piece fresh turmeric root*

1 banana

2 tablespoons Acai powder**

2 tablespoons raw hemp seeds*** (soaked for 5 hours and rinsed

2 tablespoons Chia seeds (soaked overnight and rinsed) ****

*Turmeric has a history of use in herbal remedies.

**Acai powder is a rich source of anti-oxidants

***Hemp powder is one of the richest plant sources of protein, omega fatty acids, and fiber

****Chia reduces food cravings helps hydration, lowers blood pressure and is rich in Omega 3 as well as being a brain and good cholesterol booster.

Directions

Juice the first five ingredients, and then put into the blender. Add the remaining ingredients and blend slowly. If you don't have a juicer, put all the ingredients in the blender except for the lime, ginger, and turmeric; blend. Peel the ginger, lime, and turmeric, and blend until smooth.

Chapter 6- 10 Fat Busting Fruit & Juice Recipes

Today, more than ever before, a high percentage of what we eat consists of heavily processed foods. These foods, while inexpensive to produce and purchase, contain little to no true nutritional content. Much of what we consume today is "food like" in that it is edible and will fill your stomach, but does not provide the nutrients that your body needs to operate properly. Generally speaking, this "food" is high in refined sugars and trans-fat from unhealthy oils. Due to this lack of nutrition, individuals throughout the world have experienced what they see as uncontrollable weight gain.

Without any direction, many people turn to the most heavily advertised "solutions" like weight loss pills or miracle diets. Unfortunately, a very low number of these options truly work, and most leave the dieter feeling worse than they did before. What can be done then? The only viable option to lose weight in a healthy way is to reintroduce the nutrient rich foods that our bodies are designed to take in. To be more specific: vegetables and fruits! The problem is that with our busy lives, it can be extremely difficult to find the time to make and eat a salad three times in a day. This is where juicing comes in. Juicing is a quick and easy way to provide your body with a plethora of nutrients that will help it thrive! No need to take the time to chew and swallow an entire salad. You can easily drink up 5-10 fruits and vegetables in a minute or two.

Below are the some great fat busting fruit and juice recipes, from tastiest to most powerful! If using a conventional blender, cut up each ingredient listed and add water so that it will blend properly. If you are using a modern juicer, whole vegetables and fruits are fine. For the best possible quality and health, purchase organic fruits and vegetables when possible.

Sweet Fruit

A perfect way to dip your toes into the world of juicing without shocking your taste buds! Kale is a staple ingredient for juicing because it is a super-food that is loaded with nutrients!

Ingredients

1 apple
½ lime
½ mango
2-3 oz pineapple
2-4 leaves of steamed kale
2 cucumbers
1-3 pieces of celery

Directions

Place ingredients in a blender and blend until consistency is smooth then serve.

Total Juice

Well rounded with a great mix of fruits and vegetables

Ingredients

1 apple
2-3 oz pineapple
½ banana
3-5 leaves of steamed kale
2 cucumbers
1-3 pieces of celery
2 small or medium carrots

Directions

Place ingredients in a blender and blend until consistency is smooth then serve.

Power Punch

More vegetables and less fruit mean less sugar content. Added Chia seeds are high in fiber and help to detox your intestines.

Ingredients

1 apple
2-3 oz pineapple
5-6 leaves of steamed kale
2 ½ cucumbers
3 pieces of celery
1 tsp Chia seeds

2 small or medium carrots

Directions

Place ingredients in a blender and blend until consistency is smooth then serve.

Green Attack

Lots of green vegetables here for a nutrient kick! It is not very sweet but more potent than the previous recipes.

Ingredients

½ apple
1 oz watermelon
5-6 leaves of steamed kale
1-3 leaves of steamed spinach
2 ½ cucumbers
3-4 pieces of celery
1 tsp chia seeds
1 tsp spirulina

Directions

Place ingredients in a blender and blend until consistency is smooth then serve.

Orange Attack

Carrots are rich in beta-carotene, a powerful antioxidant that converts to vitamin A once ingested.

Ingredients

3-5 small or medium carrots
½ mango
½ orange
2 leaves of kale

Directions

Place ingredients in a blender and blend until consistency is smooth then serve.

Fiber Cleanse

These high fiber ingredients will cleanse your intestines and colon of waste that was left behind.

Ingredients

½ apple
½ orange
3-5 leaves of steamed kale
1-3 leaves of steamed spinach
2 pieces of celery
2 tsp of Chia seeds
2 tsp spirulina
1 tsp wheat grass

Directions

Place ingredients in a blender and blend until consistency is smooth then serve.

Ginger Kick

Ginger is an amazing super-food that promotes a number of healthy processes in the body. Nausea, clogged sinuses, cramps, and nutrient absorption are just a few things that ginger aids in.

Ingredients

½ apple
½ mango
4 leaves of steamed kale
½ inch slice of ginger
2 cucumbers
1 tsp Chia seeds

Directions

Place ingredients in a blender and blend until consistency is smooth then serve.

Veggie Delight

Even more vegetables here and less fruit!

Ingredients

½ lime

1 oz watermelon
3 leaves of steamed kale
2 cucumbers
3 pieces of celery
2 small or medium carrots
1 tsp spirulina

Directions

Place ingredients in a blender and blend until consistency is smooth then serve.

Vitality

This is pretty potent. This combination will have you wanting to run a marathon!

Ingredients

1oz pineapple
1oz watermelon
4 leaves of steamed kale
3 small or medium carrots
2 tsp wheat grass
½ avocado
3 pieces of celery
½ inch slice of ginger
1 tsp Chia seeds

Directions

Place ingredients in a blender and blend until consistency is smooth then serve.

Superman

The doomsday smoothie! If you can handle this smoothie, you will feel absolutely amazing! If #9 made you run a marathon, this shake will make you want to take on Mike Tyson in his prime!

Ingredients

½ apple
5 leaves of steamed kale
2 cucumbers
3 small or medium carrots
4 pieces of celery
1 inch slice of ginger
2 tsp Chia seeds
2 tsp spirulina
2 tsp wheat grass
½ avocado

Directions

Place ingredients in a blender and blend until consistency is smooth then serve.

If you have never juiced before, I strongly urge you to try out these recipes! You may notice that some ingredients like kale, celery, and cucumber are listed in almost every recipe. This is because they are high nutrients and water, which causes your body to operate much more efficiently, and in turn prompts your body to shed unneeded fat that is being stored. Feel free to experiment with these recipes to fit your liking.

Just be aware that while fruits do contain vitamins and minerals like vegetables, they are also high in sugar and excess sugar in the body (more than is burnt off) is converted into fat. One thing to remember when embarking on a new dietary journey is that consistency is absolutely essential! If you decide that you are going to make one of these smoothies only one time per week, do not expect to see much change in your body. In order to lose weight and truly feel healthy and alive, you must stick to what you start. If you cannot afford to make a smoothie every day, try for every other day. Just remember to keep it consistent and you will see results!!

Chapter 7- 10 Fat Busting Detox Juice Recipes

Tropical Twist

Ingredients

½ cup cubed pineapple
¼ cup coconut water
1 chopped apple
2 tablespoon lime juice
1 cup spinach leaves
5 ice cubes

Directions

Measure all ingredients except the ice cubes into the blender and process until smooth. Next, add the ice cubes. Process until the ice cubes have been integrated into the mixture to create your desired consistency. These thinning ingredients will power your day and fight tough deposits of fat.

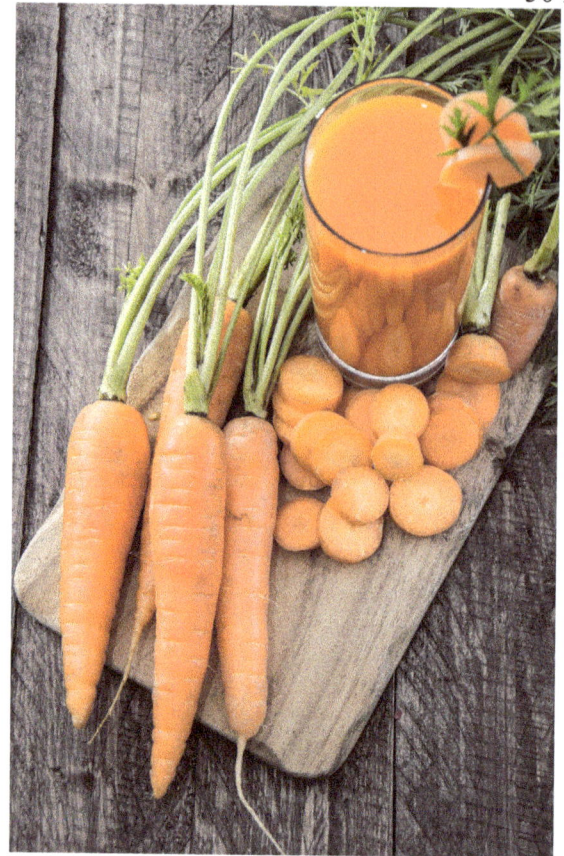

Amplified Carrot Juice

Ingredients

1 inch piece of fresh ginger
1 large red apple
10 large carrots
1 c fresh cherries
Pinch of salt

Directions

To make this recipe, use a high power juicer. Carefully feed the items one at a time through the juicer until all of the items have been processed. Depending on your desired level of sweetness, you may want to add one more small apple or an additional small handful (about 1/3 cup) of fresh cherries. Another way to sweeten the juice is to add a teaspoon or so of granulated sugar, or the healthier option, some honey for a more natural sweetener. Even though this recipe is sweet, don't let it fool you. It is jam packed with ingredients that will keep slim you down.

The Potassium and Iron Boost

Ingredients

2 large bananas, peeled and split into pieces
1½ cup spinach
1 large apple
¼ cup orange juice
5 ice cubes

Directions

Using a blender, mix together all of the ingredients except the ice cubes until they are well combined. Next, add the ice cubes. Process the mixture carefully in pulses until the ice has been broken up in small pieces evenly throughout the juice. The spinach and bananas will provide you with your iron and potassium requirements for the day, all in one simple juice.

Sweet and Spicy Apple Cider

Ingredients

6 large apples (Gala apples are preferred)
1 tablespoon honey
2 tablespoon fresh squeezed orange juice
2 teaspoon cinnamon
1 teaspoon ginger
1 teaspoon nutmeg
½ teaspoon red chili powder

Directions

Using a juicer, process all of the apples in a cup. Next, pour the apple juice into a medium sized saucepan. Heat the apples with the honey and orange juice over medium heat. Next, add the cinnamon, ginger, nutmeg, and red chili powder to the saucepan. Allow the juice to come to a boil, and then simmer the juice for about 5 minutes to allow the flavors to thoroughly combine. Once finished, allow the cider to cool for several minutes before serving as it will be hot. Serve the cider in mugs. Honey, cinnamon, and red chili powder are all substances known to help you burn more calories. Red chili powder and cinnamon are known for cleansing and rejuvenating the system as well.

Red Power Juice

Ingredients

1 full beet root, cut into slices
1 inch piece of ginger
2 large carrots

1 large apple

2 thick slices peeled, and de-seeded cucumbers

Directions

To complete this recipe, use your juice to carefully process the slices of beets. Follow the beets with ginger, the carrots, apple, and finally the cucumber slices. This drink will help detox your body by providing plenty of fiber that is particularly abundant in the beets. The ginger helps act as a natural healer and can help one feel calm and collected which is essential in any journey to well-being, detoxification, and weight loss.

Acai Berry Blaster

Ingredients

¼ cup acai berry puree

1½ cup strawberries

¾ cup blueberries

1 small banana, peeled and split into pieces

1 tablespoon pure cacao powder

1 cup non-dairy milk

Directions

Carefully add all of the ingredients into the blender and pulse on medium powder until all of the ingredients have been combined and the mixture is smooth. Drinking this juice provides loads of health benefits. Acai has recently received a great deal of attention in the media for being one of healthiest foods found on earth. Acai berries can fight immune problems and really strengthen the entire immune system. Acai also provide help regulating the digestive system and can help burn fat, both of these benefits aid in the process of fat loss.

Gulp of Green Goodness

Ingredients

1½ cups shredded kale
½ cucumber, peeled and chopped with seeds removed
¼ cup freshly squeezed orange juice
2 small green apples, cored and chopped
5 cubes ice

Directions

Add the kale, cucumber, orange juice, and apples to the blender. Pulse together all of the ingredients until the mixture is smooth. Then, add the ice and continue to pulse until the ice has been disturbed to create a slushy texture. The main ingredient in this recipe, kale, is a powerful food that provided copious amounts of fiber, iron, and other essential vitamins and nutrients, combined with other ingredients of good goodness, this mixture is an indulgence in health.

Amazing Avocado Juice

Ingredients

1 medium avocado, pitted and peeled
3 medium peaches, pitted and peeled
¼ cup Greek yogurt

Directions

Slice up the peaches and avocado and throw them in the blender. Add the yogurt to the blender. Process together the three ingredients in a blender. This incredible combination is not only delicious, but provides many essential nutrients. The avocado is jam-packed with essential oils and fats. Despite popular belief, these healthy fats are actually an important key in fat loss.

Blueberry, Spinach, and Avocado Blend

Ingredients

1 cup shredded spinach
1 small avocado, pitted and peeled
1 cup frozen blueberries

Directions

Add all of the ingredients to the blender and process until the smoothie is of the desired consistency. Spinach provides iron, the avocado healthy fats, and the blueberries are full of antioxidants. All of these elements are important for body detoxification.

Purple Dandelion Smoothies

Ingredients

l cup blueberries

1 cup cherries

2 Medjool Dates* (seed removed)

Bunch of dandelions to taste

Add spinach if needed to make up for the greens (optiona1)

2 cups of water

1 tablespoon hemp hearts (optional)

Directions

Mix all ingredients in a high powered blender like the Vitamix or your normal kitchen blender and process until desired consistency.

Medjool Dates are a type of tree fruit originating in the Middle East and North Africa and other desert-like regions around the world. They have a sweet taste and juicy flesh even when they are dried.

To minimize slightly bitter taste of dandelion greens, pick before flowers have blossomed. Also the use of strong tasting fruit to go with the greens helps to overcome the sometimes bitter flavor of the greens.

ABOUT THE AUTHOR

Amy Zulpa learned the art of juicing from her mother and grandmother and has never forgotten it since. Of course she was not too keen on the taste of some of the vegetable juices that they made but when she became an adult, she began to appreciate the nutrients that they provided for the body. She has a real passion for any food that will make the body healthier and as such she was is an avid promoter of the juicing process.

Amy has written quite a number of books, each focused on various aspects of regaining health and wellness and one of her latest publications focuses on the benefits of juicing.

www.ingramcontent.com/pod-product-compliance
Ingram Content Group UK Ltd.
Pitfield, Milton Keynes, MK11 3LW, UK
UKHW050419240426
12048UKWH00014B/709